HOW TO BEAT IBS

"From Crippling Pain To Pain Free"

By Olivia Lucs

Copyright 2013 Olivia Lucs

PREFACE

I wanted to share my story with you because I thought there was no hope for me and I struggled to find resources in my daily battle with IBS. There were no step by step guides to heal your body and get rid of this debilitating illness. I wanted to get better desperately as my life crumbled around me.

IBS can single handledly ruin your life and I have yet to meet anyone without IBS that truly understands how excruciating and life altering the condition can be. Such is the trauma, that IBS sufferers have an increased risk of suicide that is two to four times higher than those individuals without IBS symptoms. In fact, IBS sufferers have a suicide risk that is even higher that those with medically diagnosed and potentially life threatening Inflammatory Bowel Disease (IBD) such as Chron's disease.

People with IBS suffer extraordinarily and are forced to live a greatly reduced quality of life, which is amplified when family, friends, and doctors don't think their suffering is legitimate.

I felt both despair and isolation as I was confined to life on the couch unable to manage my pain and outlook on life. Doctors had told me that IBS was 'incurable' and my life, as I knew it came to a grinding halt.

IBS had a devastating effect on everything from my career to my social life to my emotional mindset. I searched endlessly for healing success stories during my struggle to give me hope and to know that I was not condemned to a life of hell. Had I known then what I know now, my experience would have been much easier to live through and I would have recovered a lot quicker. I promised myself the second I was better, I would share my story and try to help other sufferers by showing that it can be done. It is a sorry state of affairs when all you want and pray for is a pain free existence. It really does make you strip back your life and get back to basics by appreciating the simple things in life that others take for granted.

IBS is a misunderstood illness and the general population has heard it in passing, thinking of it more or less as a stomach ache. It is much more than that, and can cause devastating pain akin to the "suffering of a cancer patient", as one of my previous specialists had noted. Society is just uninformed. I used to be one of those people, until I lived it every day and it ruled my life. I believe the medical community is starting to acknowledge the extent and severity of IBS, but there is still a long road ahead. I am hopeful that a cure is achievable one day in the not too distant future.

Although my experience with IBS may be different to yours, I want you to know that I understand what it is like to experience chronic, indescribable abdominal pain that no one around you can comprehend, and I sympathise unconditionally. I understand what it feels like to have no hope for the future as this illness has an incomprehensible and dramatic effect on every aspect of your life.

I hope that sharing what I have learned along the way can help you get to a better place in managing and, ultimately eliminating pain from your life. There is light at the end of the tunnel and you will be stronger for it. Don't give up even if you can not imagine one more day of IBS. I didn't. You can dramatically improve your health and overcome your uphill battle with this condition. I am living proof that it can be done so never give up even when you think the world is against you and everyone is telling you to just accept it. Reclaim your life and get rid of IBS forever so you can live a normal life, a life without pain, a life that you deserve.

MY STORY

2010 and I thought I was going to die. Gripping, indescribable pain churned through my body as though there was an alien trying to force its way out of me. Life as I knew it would never be the same. And I was never going to be the same.

For 28 years I had lived a healthy, active and normal lifestyle. I was a happy, positive person who loved their life. Having literally just returned from an amazing vacation with my partner to Mexico, I found myself sitting on the couch with ridiculous gurgling sounds emanating from below my belly and pain that I could not ascribe to any particular organ. For the first time in my life, I became conscious of my insides at work and wondered what on Earth was going on. There was no way I could possibly foresee what was going to happen to me and my journey to hell began that night.

I went to the doctor next day, who once informed of my travelling holiday gave me an obligatory course of the antibiotic Flagyl, which would kill any bad bug in my body. My partner had the runs while we were in Mexico so the doctor put two and two together and assumed I had picked up a nasty bug. No blood or stool tests were ordered. Little did I know, that Flagyl would also kill off all the good bacteria in my body too.

A week rolled on with no improvement so I saw another doctor. This time I was given Doxycycline and a battery of tests were ordered. Nothing changed, I still had rumbling and random stabbing pains, like razor blades on my left side. A week after that, another doctor, another course of antibiotics, followed by another "we can't find anything wrong with you". Times this by 50 and that would be close to the times I repeated this cycle of hell. I felt like I was talking to a brick wall. I listened and trusted the doctor's advice. Of course, they would know best, right? Meanwhile in the back of my mind, I knew that all these antibiotics were making me feel worse but clinging desperately to hope, I thought that maybe the next one would help. All the while, my pain became more and more severe. Coupled with constipation, excruciating cramps, occasional diarrhoea, and waves of abdominal pain, living became unbearable and my life non-existent.

And so continued the next 6 months, multiple doctors, expensive specialists and perfect test results. I was perfect healthily they told me, yet continued to feel sicker and sicker, until bam, excruciating pain became my every minute and it riddled my body. Burning, ripping, churning, violent contractions, that would keep me up, all day, all night, with no respite. It felt like my insides were being ripped apart and I would cry out in pain. I had become a prisoner in my body. And what's more, no one understood or seemed to care. I just had a stomach ache right?

IBS is so much more than that. Staying awake for 24 hours a day, night after night, in gripping pain and with no one able to give you a plausible explanation, has an extraordinary effect on your mind, spirit and body. All three disintegrated to the lowest form.

I changed my diet and tried to adopt the FODMAP diet, and realised some food such as dairy and oatmeal gave me instant painful contractions. It was difficult to stick to the diet and I did not follow it religiously. I took swags of vitamins and supplements, and increased my fibre whilst taking movicol to ensure regularity. Nothing seemed to work and I reverted back to old eating habits. I felt disillusioned with the advice from the medical industry and online resources. I was told just to accept my condition, but how could I. This was no life. I felt like a lost cause.

I became paralysed with pain unable to function at all and became couch ridden dosed upon a cocktail of pain killers. Doubled over in teeth clenching pain, I finally surrendered to pain relief. This coming from a person who had always prided themselves on being a pinnacle of health and who had vehemently steered clear of medicating themselves. The pain killers dulled the pain but never completely eradicated it and what's more I felt drugged and out of it for days. They had become a coping mechanism as my brain struggled to comprehend why this was happening to me and if this would become my life?

My nights were spent wide awake stressed that i would have to call in sick to work, rolling around in pain for 8 hours straight with zero sleep. My partner was at first sympathetic, for a week, and then would just yell at me, telling me to take pain killers, or shut up and let them get some sleep.

My life was falling apart, being completely incapacitated by pain, which no one could explain. After numerous trips to the ER department, I was subjected to multiple blood tests, stool tests, upper and lower abdominal ultrasounds, abdominal x-rays, CT scans, a hida scan for gallbladder functionality and an MRI of the small bowel. By my sixth visit, having never once in 28 years been in hospital, the doctors were dismissive and did not care to deal with me. The emergency department were just happy to delve out pain medication, usually in the form of endone and morphine, which would mask the symptoms with the pain returning with a vengeance when I returned home.

During one of my stays in hospital, I even had a visit from the registered psychologist who wanted to assess me. His diagnosis was that I should be put on anti depressants. This just made me mad, I wanted help not more medication and excuses. No pain would equal immediate happiness! Then the dreaded Irritable Bowel Syndrome (IBS) diagnosis was bounced around, basically a term given when all other 'serious' conditions had been eliminated from diagnosis. It is a functional disorder where bowels looked okay to the eye, but for some unknown reason, they were not functioning as they did before and had become hypersensitive to pain. Normal stretching of the bowel to allow for gas would now cause pain. I knew this to be partially true when I woke up inadvertently during a colonoscopy to incredible pain. I screamed out as they circumnavigated through a bend in my large bowel. But IBS is a loosely thrown around diagnosis when they have no idea, and it is down played like a headache. Well you have labour pains 24 hours a day, 7 days a week, and you see how you feel!

No one could give me answers and some even had the indecency of suggesting that it was all in my head. I found myself breaking down all the time telling my parents that I wanted to die, that "this was no life", and that I could not live the rest of my life like this. My partner, on the other hand, would just roll their eyes and told me they were "sick of hearing about it", and "shut up, and get a job", I was a positive person, who used to smile all the time and this had been wiped from my life in its entirety. I could not enjoy any activities that I did previously. How could I if I was constant pain?

It did not take long until I was fired from my job, because they needed "someone that would turn up". To some extent, this relieved some pressure off me, because now I could concentrate on getting better. My life, however, continued to crumble.

I spent all my savings on doctors and specialists, and racked up considerable debt. I had 3 colonoscopies and 3 gastroscopies in total over the course of a year and a half. Each with a different specialist. Out of sheer desperation, I had lied to each of them saying it was my first time, hoping that they would find something, anything to fix. Different doctors, different emergency departments but still the same result. "Sorry we have never seen any one like you – you just have a severe case of IBS".

I proceeded to look down different avenues to explain the pain, seeing gynaecologists to rule out any gynaecological abnormalities. I had a laparoscopy, primarily to look for endometriosis, and results for this came back entirely normal except for that fact that the surgeon noted that my small intestine was bouncing around like a snake and he had never seen anything like it! I took this information to the gastroenterologists who of course dismissed it, as gynaecologists know nothing about their field (no they just had a first hand account and saw it with their own eyes!) and it was probably just responding to gas used during the procedure.

Losing hope fast, I did find one gastroenterologist who was willing to investigate this finding further and gave me a capsule endoscopy where by you swallow a tiny camera and it takes hundreds of images as it passes through your small bowel to check for abnormalities. This test too proved to be normal. I was now resigned to the fact that I had IBS, an incurable condition I was told, that I had to live with for the rest of my life.

Feeling that my life was slipping away from me, I took it upon myself to google obsessively and resolved that if doctors would not help me, I would. I was house bound and had shut myself off from the world. How could I call my friends and tell them that I was still in severe pain and wanted to die? Who would believe me, no one would understand. As I trawled through the net, I found similar stories of despair and for the first time in this horrific journey, I had found some solace. There were people out there like me. I was not alone any more, and what is more, was that they understood how unrelenting and soul crushing IBS was. Unless you had chronic, debilitating pain, there is no way you could fathom what it does to you as a person and to your life. These fellow IBS sufferers did not have a mental condition, nor were they desperate for attention. Tears would roll down my face as I read their stories – no, they were 'normal' human beings, like me.

My partner had become disgusted with me and would call me lazy and pathetic, tell me that there was nothing wrong with me, to get a job, and that they were going out to have some fun with "normal" people. A ten year relationship had disintegrated into countless tirades of abuse and eye rolls. Your partner is supposed to be your pillar of strength and you are supposed to be able to lean on them in times of need. This is the person I thought I was going to spend the rest of my life with, instead they became the enemy. Time and time again, I would be dumped outside the hospital door and told to stay there until I sorted myself out. It was at this low point, whilst I spent two weeks alone and helpless in a hospital bed, that I told myself the second I was better and stronger, I would leave the relationship. At one point, I even had my appendix taken out, because I thought it would show my partner that I was trying to get better. It did for a day, until the unrelenting pain came back, and then I was just a "loser" again.

IBS, something incurable, something you have for life. My life as I knew it, was over. I was dumped, fittingly by text, after ten years together, had been fired from my job and spent every day lying on the couch restricted by severe pain. The only thing I had, apart from the support of my parents, was the internet and my friend Doctor Google. I spent days, weeks, months, on there, googling every similar story, noting any medication, herbal tincture, treatments that I could try, that I could possibly try. Even if there was a 1% chance, I would do it. I trawled through the net endlessly searching for stories where IBS sufferers had eliminated their pain. I copped a lot of "stop wasting your time on the internet", and "you're becoming obsessed with google", but as only an IBS sufferer would know, hearing stories of fellow sufferers and searching for hope of relief, is an absolute must when living this horrendous condition and I make no excuses for living on the computer. The fundamental instinct to live ultimately kicked in and I wanted my life back desperately.

I stumbled across the badbugs.com website and made an appointment at the Centre of Digestive Diseases. The badbugs website is a brilliant resource that thinks "outside the box" of normal IBS theory and it helped me identify a secondary bowel infection, that is, parasite, that was not picked up in order testing by general practitioners. I had a liquid fixative stool test which I went on to learn was a much more accurate form of testing for parasites, and was angry that I was not given this option prior during my numerous visits to doctors. Subsequently, I tested positive to the bug Diaentomeba Fragilis, and was given the specific protocol treatment of secnidazole and doxycycline. I was incredibly hopeful that my pain would come to an end, but tests confirming that the bug had been nuked did not unfortunately relay a pain free existence. It was, however, possible that was now I was dealing with post infectious IBS.

Hopes dashed I saw numerous natural practitioners, purchased many home remedies which did nothing but empty my purse and make me gag. I even resorted to spiritual healing for the soul, and went to countless sessions of chanting. Whilst I can not say that my condition improved, I did feel better emotionally after each session because these people showed empathy and kindness towards me, spurring me on to not give up.

I had a strange encounter with an alternative practitioner who at one point put a tennis racquet on my head and plugged it into some electromagnet device which would Channel energy into areas of my body that were not operating to full capacity. Although it was frustrating, it did provide light entertainment. Another encounter with a different practitioner had me connected to a Russian machine that would read the frequency of each body organ and not only indicate if there was a problem, but also offer a solution. Unfortunately my ears and kidney were the only issues, neither of which have ever caused me troubles. Another healer saw spiders inside my body and told me to drink whiskey. I then knew it was up to me to change my life.

I researched small bowel bacterial overgrowth (SIBO) as being a prominent cause of IBS, and tried rifaximin prior to testing. Rifaximin, a non-absorbic antibiotic, was recently shown over a 10 day period to result in a dramatic improvement in bloating and overall symptoms of IBS. This course had no impact on my IBS symptoms, in fact I suffered considerable diarrhoea, and the subsequent breath test for SIBO that I undertook at a later stage came back negative.

Somehow through all of this, I met my new partner and was upfront about my condition straight away. They were patient and understanding, and willing to help me get through this, a stark contrast to the former, and I had known them only for a matter of weeks. Although it was tough and certainly tested the relationship at times, support is an undeniable factor in the healing process. No one can possibly understand chronic pain, unless they have suffered and been through it, but empathy can empower you with the mental capacity to go on. I believe the body is meant to heal itself but this requires the coordination and stability of multiple environmental factors, and of course, consistency and discipline.

I started looking after myself, initiating a strict diet and regime of well researched vitamins and supplements. I consistently ate a high protein, lean meat such as chicken/ fish and steamed vegetables, minimising my intake of carbohydrates. I avoided dairy, sugar, fatty and processed foods like the plague. I started drinking loads of herbal teas and filtered water throughout each day. I would apply a combined oil of peppermint, fennel and Rosemary to my abdomen each night. I took endep at night to relax the smooth muscle of the GI tract and to ensure I had a good nights sleep required to heal the body. For the first time, I was getting successive hours of sleep. I completely steered clear of antibiotics and I started going to regular sauna sessions to detox and found a wonderful acupuncturist who was able to give me treatments that were not only relaxing but provided pain relief. I increased my exercise levels gradually. And guess what?

I actually started feeling a slight improvement. I began experiencing pain free hours and for the first time, I could finally see the fruits from my hard work. Yes as ridiculous as it sounds, a pain free hour for me, was somewhat of a milestone and something to smile about. These pain free hours then became pain free days, and gradually the time between my attacks grew longer and longer. The pain gradually dissipated. I knew that finally, and thankfully, I was on the path to recovery.

There were undoubtedly hiccups along the way like when I ate something that had dairy, or was loaded with excessive sugar, or was too fatty. This would then initiate an attack that would be set me back and I would have to start with the basics again. But these attacks became shorter in duration and had lessened in intensity, as my body had become healthier and stronger. Eventually these attacks became non-existent, and I could eat whatever I want without invoking a painful digestive reaction.

Each day when I wake I make sure to be thankful for feeling healthy and having a normal life. I can not help but smile. Some times I even have to pinch myself that this is my reality now, such was the emotional trauma that I had endured. I survived and I was stronger person for it.

The importance is to have a solid foundation. Without it, it is near impossible to bounce back and overcome IBS. After all it is a combination of mind, body and soul that will lead to your recovery. Ditch the negative environment and mindset, do adopt a strict, basic diet and ensure you take the correct vitamins and supplements. Above all, be consistent, don't cheat. Know that your body is healing and tell yourself every day that you are getting better and better. You need to believe and have patience and dedication. It takes time but the body is designed to heal and rebalance itself.

WHAT IS IBS?

Irritable Bowel Syndrome (IBS) is a common physical disorder of the gastrointestinal tract (GI) that causes recurrent upper and lower symptoms. The normal rhythm of the muscular contractions in the digestive tract become irregular and uncoordinated disrupting the movement of food and waste, and trapping gas and stool. This causes abdominal pain, bloating, mucous in stools, constipation and diarrhoea, however not all patients with the same diagnosis are created equal.

Other terms for IBS include 'spastic colon' or 'irritable colon'.

IBS is not a disease, it is a functional disorder where a group of symptoms occur together, and is characterized as a brain-gut dysfunction. The severity of the pain can vary from mild to severe from person to person, and also in duration, from intermittent to constant. Triggers in one person may be different to triggers in another.

The Rome criteria are the current standard for diagnosis of IBS and it presumes the absence of a structural or biochemical cause. IBS is diagnosed when a person has had abdominal pain/ discomfort at least 3 times a month for the last 3 months without any other explanation for the pain. The pain may occur with a change in stool frequency or consistency or be relieved by a bowel motion.

Other Common Symptoms include:

- Abdominal pain or cramping that is often relieved by passing gas or faeces.
- Alternating diarrhoea and constipation.
- A sensation that the bowels are not fully emptied after passing a motion.
- Abdominal bloating.
- Mucous present in stools - a clear liquid produced by intestines to coat and protect tissues in GI tract
- Nausea

IBS does not present the same way in all people so IBS is classified according to the primary symptom that patients experience:

- IBS with constipation (IBS-C)

- IBS with diarrhoea (IBS-D)

- IBS with alternation constipation and diarrhoea (IBS-A)

The classifications assist in providing specific types of treatment for each category.

While food sensitivities, and small bowel overgrowth, are known to cause IBS symptoms, there may be other causes such as parasitic infection, mineral deficiencies, lack of enzymes, hormonal imbalance and emotional stress.

Up to 20% of the population suffer some form of IBS. Women are 2 to 3 times more likely to be diagnosed with IBS then men.

Abnormalities in gut flora through infection, antibiotic use etc are believed to lead to inflammation thus causing altered bowel function. There are 500 species of bugs and one hundred trillion bacterial in your gut ecosystem and they need to be in balance for you to be healthy.

Research has shown there may be brain – gut signal problems with abnormalities in the gastrointestinal nervous system causing greater than normal discomfort or hypersensitivity when your abdomen stretches from gas or stool. Poorly coordinated signals between the brain and the intestines can make your body overreact to changes that normally occur in the digestive process. This overreaction in the form of spasms or sudden, strong muscle contractions can cause pain, diarrhoea or constipation through abnormal movements of the colon and small intestines. .

Research indicates that the neurotransmitter serotonin may be key in altering the make-up of nerve cells in the bowel causing a change in pain sensation and bowel function.

Whilst IBS can be disabling and devastating, it does not cause permanent damage to the bowel and does not lead to the development of serious conditions such as colitis and cancer.

STEP BY STEP GUIDE TO HEALING

Whilst each person with IBS is different and has a different story, I believe the following are key elements to healing and becoming pain free. I wasted a lot of time, chopping and changing, searching through online resources, and not sticking to a plan. I could not find a centralized resource that gave me a step by step guide to controlling my IBS and swore to myself that once I was better, I would culminate all the knowledge that I had gathered along my journey and draft a guide to help others. Even if you are in pain and feel like you cant do anything, please try and start now. Your body needs time to heal so don't procrastinate any longer.

Essentially you need to remove the bugs, yeast, parasites, irritating foods; replace missing enzymes; provide nutritional support to repair the gut; and replenish a healthy bacterial balance within your system through probiotics.

Follow the steps below consistently and diligently, and you should feel better within a few months and get your life back. If you notice an improvement in your pain over the 3 months, but it has not been completely eradicated, stick to the below regime for at least another 3 – 6 months to ensure adequate healing.

1. Surround yourself by positivity

- Ditch negative relationships or any one making you feel guilty for being sick. You are doing nothing wrong and deserve emotional support and compassion. They say that you see a person's true colours during tough times and this is entirely correct. Do not suffer with IBS in silence.

- Do hang off people that tell you not to give up, tell you that you will feel better, and tell you to keep trying.

- Adopt a positive mindset. Dealing with toxic emotions can help speed up the healing process. Although it is difficult to be positive when you feel so terrible, see it as an opportunity to turn your entire life around. I managed to free myself from a terribly negative relationship and a job that I wasn't enjoying, and I am in a better place today for it. Your body is designed to heal itself, you just need to give it a chance.

- Do not be afraid to take pain killers to get you through the rough periods. I suffered unnecessarily because I did not want to mask the symptoms and to rely on medication. As a result, my mental state suffered dramatically. You can be resourceful during this time and start planning your recovery. No one deserves to be in chronic pain so use the help if required.

- Manage your stress levels as this can severely aggravate the condition and send your adrenal system into overdrive zapping your body of vital nutrients required for healing. Gentle exercises, walking, yoga, meditation, controlled breathing and relaxation techniques may assist in reducing your overall stress levels.

2. Adopt a strict diet

- Stick to the basics, eating lean meat/fish and cooked vegetables for at least 3 months. Avoid too much fruit. Have one portion of fruit maximum a day and ensure it is a low FODMAP food.

- Incorporate the FODMAP diet, but avoid raw food and fruit during this 3 month time period. After 3 months, gradually introduce raw food and fruit, noting which types to avoid according to the diet and also note which foods you have an adverse reaction to, as each person is different.

Researchers from Melbourne's Monash University in Australia have found that eating a diet low in certain carbohydrates (sugars) can help alleviate symptoms by up to 75% of IBS patients. These carbohydrates are called FODMAP for short, an acronym for Fermentable Oligosaccharides, Disaccharides, Monosaccharides, and Polyols. FODMAPS are found in many common foods such as dairy, wheat and some fruits and vegetables such as apples, onions and cauliflower.

The theory behind the diet is that by consuming certain foods which are high in FODMAP's, results in an increased volume of liquid and gas in the small and large intestine, which leads to uncomfortable symptoms such as distension, abdominal pain, diarrhoea, constipation, gas and bloating.

- Avoid having grains, dairy, chocolate, spicy and fatty foods at all times as they are irritating to the GI tract.

- Avoid sugar, which may interfere with the balance of bacteria, and creates fermentation in the bowel, which leads to the uncomfortable effects of gas and bloating.

- Avoid eating any processed food, or adding any condiments, sauces, sweeteners etc to your food.

- Try to cook at home as often as possible as home cooking is a lot healthier than eating out and makes it much easier to monitor your dietary intake. You know what is going into each meal and restaurants regularly add extra salt, fat and sugar to supplement often cheap and poor quality ingredients. Self management of your diet is critical and key to your speedy recovery.

- Try to drink at least 2 - 3 litres purified water a day to keep fibre moving smoothly through your system. Have a large glass of room temperature water upon waking and before bed. Water is essential for combatting constipation and replaces the extra fluid lost if diarrhoea is a factor.

- Limit drinks to herbal teas, and water, and avoid carbonated drinks. In addition, completely avoid alcohol, tobacco and caffeine, as they are known stimulants and irritants to the digestive tract.

Consume these teas and water regularly throughout the day and ensure that they do not have any additives such as caffeine. These teas have been proven to have a soothing effect on the gastrointestinal tract. They possess anti spasmodic qualities that will reduce intestinal spasms and relieve gas.

As with all foods, reactions may vary with each individual. Note which ones work for you and keep sipping throughout the day. I personally swear by camomile with a fresh slice of ginger, which worked best for me.

Teas to try include:

- Peppermint tea – avoid if you have reflux
- Camomile tea - has anti inflammatory properties
- Ginger tea
- Fennel tea – best for bloating and gas

Alternatively, you can take enteric coated peppermint oil capsules. The coating ensures that the oil reaches the intestine instead of breaking down in the stomach. Clinical studies have shown that they are as effective as anti-spasmodics for alleviating IBS symptoms, and do not have the side effects that prescription ati-spasmodics do (dry mouth, sleepiness, dizziness). Be cautious if you have reflux as they may trigger an episode. Contrary to popular findings, the capsules did not work for me and actually made me feel worse.

Take one capsule three times a day on an empty stomach and at least ½ hour before each meal.

- Start a food diary, listing all the food, drinks, and supplements you are taking and noting any adverse reactions. Sometimes it is hard to determine which food is causing what reaction. It may have an instant reaction or take a day or two to cause symptoms. That's why you need to keep to a basic diet at first, and then add in different foods and see if you are okay with it. I became aware every time i had dairy, I would have a severe attack but a couple of days after ingesting the food.

Testing:

1.   Try to get a test IgG food allergies and eliminate foods that tested positive for 12 weeks. Or just try an allergy elimination diet for a few weeks.

Alternatively, test yourself by eliminating the most common ford allergens for 12 weeks – dairy, gluten, yeast, eggs, corn, soy and peanuts. And then reintroduce them one by one to see if they produce any symptoms.

An elimination diet may be helpful in uncovering food sensitivities, and you may want to remove the trigger food indefinitely. Food sensitivities are more common than food allergies. Sugar was a massive trigger for me and I still limit my consumption even though I am pain free these days.

2.   Complete the fructose breath test – this test measures whether your intestines are able to digest and absorb fructose. A positive result indicates fructose malabsorption and your IBS can be brought under control by strictly following the FODMAP diet.

3. Maintain healthy eating patterns

- Eat small meals regularly throughout the day to help your digestive system establish a routine and do not overload your stomach. Avoid missing meals or leaving long gaps between eating.

- Eat your food slowly and chew. Make sure you are relaxed and sitting down. Taking time to chew means properly means that the digestive processes have already started before the food enters the stomach, and also gives the stomach time to prepare the enzymes and gastric juices needed for the foods digestion. Eating quickly can cause havoc to your digestion by not allowing your body to prepare and often causes you to swallow too much air which causes bothersome intestinal gas.

4. Find a good doctor/ specialist and stick with them, and adopt a pain management routine

- Ensure that they are supportive and open to trying new things. Ditch any doctor that thinks you are crazy, or a hypochondriac. Whilst you want second and third opinions, and must shop around, make sure that when you find a good, and reputable doctor/

specialist that you keep them. Its imperative to have an ongoing support network that you can rely on for your emotional well-being.

- The stigma attached to IBS is one of the most frustrating problems. We are not comfortable talking about the health of our digestive system and until the 1990's the medical community did not see IBS as an actual condition, rather a collection of psychosomatic symptoms. Undiagnosed and untreated, IBS can have devastating consequences, so a proper diagnosis from a healthcare professional is critical.

- For times of need only, ensure that you have a supply of pain medication handy such as anti spasmodic buscopan, and codeine for when pain is extreme. The anti spasmodic is used to relax muscles in the bladder and intestines. There are several types of anti spasmodics and they each work differently so find which one works for you – for example, mebeverine, hyoscine and peppermint oil. Even if you do not use them, it is comforting knowing that they are just in case and you do not have to be wheeled off to the emergency department every time you have debilitating pain.

- Heating pads can be soothing and research supports the use of low level continuous heat as a way to speed up pain relief.

- Whilst you must not become dependent on pain medication, pain management is essential to ensure a calm state of mind, and to allow your body to heal. Nobody deserves to be in constant pain and the stress of it can wear you down emotionally and wreak havoc on your immune system.

- If pain is constant and you are getting no relief, in addition to experiencing disrupted sleep, you may wish to try a special class of antidepressants, which have been clinically proven to increase your pain threshold. Often a last resort once other remedies have been trialled, it has been found that at low doses, certain antidepressants can help to modulate intestinal pain and regulate gut function. The brain and gut share chemicals, and 95% of serotonin is found in the gut assisting in smooth intestinal contractions. I requested the tricyclic anti-depressant Endep. I should of had this at the beginning as I lived a year without any sleep, suffering unnecessarily and impairing my own healing.

- Endep at low doses has been proven as a smooth muscle relaxant and as a pain reliever. It usually takes a month or two to work and feel the full benefits, so give it a chance. Start at 20mg per night and increase gradually by 10mg increments until there is sustained pain relief. The only side effect that I experienced was that it made me tired (which is good for a good nights rest), constipated and gave me dry mouth. These side effects were minimal considering the pain I was experiencing. I had a very positive experience with Endep in line with reviews from other IBS sufferers that I read online.

5. Have all necessary testing

Whilst sedative, pain killers and anti depressants may make life bearable, it is important to address the underlying cause of why your digestion is not working.

1. Laboratory testing:

Eliminate all other diseases that can cause similar symptoms to IBS, such as inflammatory bowel disease (IBD), STDs, diverticulitis, colorectal cancer and gynaecological conditions like endometriosis through the following testing:

- Full medical check up

- Blood test – starting with a Full Blood Count, and checking markers for Inflammatory Bowel Disease (IBD), coeliac disease, liver/kidney function tests, thyroid testing and vitamin levels to ensure nutrition is sufficient (magnesium, zinc, iron, calcium etc). Rule out anaemia, a lack of iron in the blood, which can cause gut problems. A high white blood cell count indicates that there is inflammation somewhere in the body. Testing Erythrocyte sedimentation rate (ESR) and C reactive protein (CRP) are further tests that detect inflammation. Inflammation is not symptomatic of IBS.

- Stool culture test– ensure it is a <u>liquid fixative test</u> conducted over a 3 day period, which are much better at detecting bugs. If infected have a repeat test, a month after antibiotics to ensure eradication. A sample should be tested for evidence of common bacteria, and parasites

- Faecal occult blood test - Blood in stool is not a symptom of IBS and could possibly mean IBD so must be followed up by additional testing. The test can detect bleeding from any part of the digestive tract even if it is not visible.

- Abdominal xray

- Abdominal ultrasound – upper and lower

- Ct scan of abdomen

- Colonoscopy – this test examines the inside of the colon and biopsies are taken from various sections for testing.

- Gastroscopy – this test is similar to the colonoscopy except the camera is inserted into the mouth and examines the oesophagus, stomach and the first part of the small bowel, known as the duodenum, from which biopsies are taken to test for coeliac disease or malabsorption such as lactose intolerance.

- For women – gynaecological testings such as pelvic ultrasound and laparoscopy to rule out conditions such as endometriosis which often exhibit similar pain/cramping

- STD testing

- HIDA scan – testing gallbladder functionality

- MRI of small bowel (for possible IBD)

- Capsule endoscopy (for possible IBD)

6. Eliminate all parasites and do not have any antibiotics unless there is positive testing

- The presence of secondary bowel flora infections such as Dientomeba Fragilis and some Blastocystis Hominis strains, and Clostridium Difficile need to be excluded.

- Take the antibiotic protocol specific for the bug identified and ensure you take a quality probiotic throughout the course. At least two hours, before or after the dose is taken to ensure that the good bacteria from the probiotic survives.

- Antibiotics severely disrupt the bacterial environment that exists in your body by eliminating good and bad bacteria so avoid antibiotics at all costs unless a parasite has been identified through testing. Try to focus on helping your own immune system to become stronger.

7. Get tested for Small Intestinal Bacterial Overgrowth (SIBO) and yeast overgrowth

- Small bowel bacterial overgrowth is a leading cause of IBS. Most bacteria live in the large intestine, but sometimes they move into the small intestine, which is supposed to be sterile. Eating starchy food will result in bloating as these bacteria ferment the sugars.

- Testing involves a simple breath test, which measures gas production by the bacteria. You must be off PPIs for at least a month as they give false results on the breath test.

- If positive, take a course of the non-absorbic antibiotic rifaximin, 550mg twice a day, over a 10 day course.

- Yeast overgrowth is common and caused when the good bacteria are crowded out through antibiotic use, steroids, acid blocking drugs and birth control pills. It's exacerbated by consuming sugar and alcohol.

- Diflucan can be taken as an anti-fungal. Take 100mg a day for a period of 4 weeks to kill the yeast. In addition, taking probiotics can ensure that the yeast in your system does not over grow beyond normal amounts. Yeast can be kept in check if sufficient beneficial bacteria exists.

8. Take probiotics to repopulate your digestive tract with good bacteria and avoid antibiotics

- Get a high quality probiotic with beneficial live bacteria such as VSL, or polybac 8 and try daily for 3 months to provide you with healthy gut flora. This is required to normalize gut function and improve digestion through better absorption of nutrients and synthesis of certain vitamins.

- Probiotics inhibit Candida overgrowth and are essential for a healthy immune response as 70% of the immune system is found in the intestinal tract.

- Quality probiotics offer multiple strains including Lactobacillus and Bifidobacteria, and are required to be refrigerated. Also take probiotic S Bourladii daily for 1-2 months to further normalize gut function.

- Take in the morning on an empty stomach and do not take other medication for at least 2 hours after.

- In addition to probiotics, incorporate probiotic rich foods into your diet, which include kimchi, sauerkraut, kefir, miso, and natural, unsweetened yoghurt (if dairy is not a problem for you).

- Increase the effects of probiotics by cutting out sugar.

9. Take vitamins and supplements to heal the lining of your gut

- Normally an IBS sufferers' digestive system is very weak, so supplementation will assist in strengthening and repairing these processes by reducing inflammation and healing a leaky gut.

- Leaky gut occurs when there is a break in the lining of your intestinal cells, and food proteins and bacteria are then able to leak into your bloodstream causing inflammation and an autoimmune response by aggravating your immune system. It compromises the body's ability to absorb nutrients and triggers bloating, gas, food sensitivities, cramps and fatigue.

- Leaky gut will irritate your second brain (the enteric nervous system) creating havoc that leads to an irritable bowel, an irritable bowel and other systemic issues including arthritis, autoimmunity, allergy and more.

- Leaky gut can be caused by sensitivity to common food allergens like gluten or dairy, by taking drugs such as nonsteroidal anti-inflammatory pills (NSAIDS), cytotoxic drugs and antibiotics, and through excessive alcohol intake.

Vitamins and Supplements:

- Take the following vitamins and supplements to speed up your recovery:

1. Fish oil – to reduce gut inflammation. Take 3 times a day with meals.

2. Multivitamin – to provide broad nutritional support. Take once in the morning.

3. Zinc – helps with digestive enzymes. Zinc carnosine supports the digestive tract and speeds up healing. Take 3 times a day with meals.

4. Evening primrose oil (GLA) – balances hormones. Lots of women notice that IBS symptoms are worse just before their periods, which may have to do with the pattern of hormonal fluctuation in the second half of the cycle. Take one with a meal.

5. L Glutamine – Glutamine is an essential amino acid that is anti-inflammatory and necessary for the growth and repair of your intestinal lining. L Glutamine protects and coats your cell walls, which effectively repels irritants.

Take one teaspoon (5g) on an empty stomach before bed and one teaspoon when you wake up.

6. Liquorice Root (DGL) – it improves acid production in the stomach and balances cortisol levels, while it maintains the mucosal lining of the stomach and the duodenum.

Take a tablet before each meal.

6. Aloe Vera Juice – is healing to the digestive tract. Take one teaspoon in the morning.

7. Turmeric – can help ease digestive complaints through its anti-inflammatory properties and its ability to block abnormal muscle contractions in the gut.

Take 500mg once a day.

8. Quercetin – has anti-inflammatory histamine blocking properties, which stabilises mast cells and reduces the release of histamine common in food sensitivities. It helps heal leaky gut by creating tight junction proteins.

Take 500mg 3 x daily with food.

8. Digestive Enzymes – often there is an inadequate secretion of digestive enzymes in IBS sufferers so using broad spectrum enzymes will aid in breaking down your food while your gut is healing. When the food has digested, it allows the body to fully absorb the nutrients that are available. In addition, bloating and gas are minimised, since the food is properly digested before it reaches the small intestine.

Take ½ hour before meals to enhance digestion and normalize bowel function.

10. Take a fibre supplement

This is essential and feeds healthy bacteria. It can help reduce abdominal pain, cramping and gas. The recommended minimum fibre intake for adults is 15 to 25 grams daily.

- A soluble fibre base is the key and can be achieved through regular consumption of a fibre supplement and soluble fibre foods like rice, pasta, potatoes and white bread. Soluble fibre should account for a third of the recommended fibre intake.

Soluble fibre soothes and regulates the digestive tract by ensuring a smooth film around the stool to allow for ease of bowel movements. It absorbs excess water in the colon and keeps the GI muscles stretched gently around a full colon, allowing muscles to easily grip during peristaltic contractions. Soluble fibre will stabilise the GI contractions that are going haywire with IBS and causing pain, and will normalize bowel function from either extreme of constipation or diarrhoea.

Insoluble fibre is also necessary but should be treated with caution. It includes foods like raw fibrous veggies, salad greens, unpeeled fruit. It aids in creating bulk in the stool and assists in the cleansing of the walls of the intestines, however can cause violent GI spasms that can be very painful and seize up the colon muscles.

- Take a fibre supplement each day starting with two tablespoons of Benefiber (or alternative such as Fibercon) and gradually increasing the dose to ensure regularity. Avoid metamucil and Fybogel (psyllium) if you have problems with gas and bloating, as they will only exacerbate the problem.

- If you have IBS C, mix with over-the-counter non stimulant type laxatives such as movicol/miralax. Try to steer clear of harsh laxatives that your body can become dependent on. Movicol is an osmotic laxative that is a gentle alternative to harsh laxatives. It works by drawing water into the stool resulting a softer stool and inducing more frequent bowel movements. Take one sachet each night before going to bed to keep the bowels moving and to ensure regular bowel movements in the morning.

- Gradually increase your fibre supplement dosage to four tablespoons a day and supplement with Gas X (simethicone) to cope with additional gas created by the increased fibre until your body adjusts the increased levels.

- You must ensure that you are consuming lots of water or herbal teas to allow the soluble fibre to normalize your bowel function. Water combines with fibre in the intestine to make your stools bulkier and easier to pass through your digestive system, and it rehydrates you if you have diarrhoea.

11. Use Iberogast

- This german concoction of clinically proven herbs manufactured by Steigerwald is used for IBS and functional dyspepsia. It has been shown to normalize intestinal tone reducing spasm and improving gut function. It can also be used for heartburn, bloating, cramping and abdominal pain.

- The all natural, liquid formulation of nine herbs was developed in Germany in 1961 and acts as a prokinetic. It is a mixture of extracts from bitter candyfruit (Iberis amara), angelica root (Angelicae radix), milk thistle fruit (Silybi mariani fructus), celandine herb (Chelidonii herba), caraway fruit (Carvi fructus), liquorice root (Liquiritiae radix), peppermint herb (Menthae piperitae folium), balm leaf (Melissae folium), and chamomile flower (Matricariae flos).

- Mix approx 20 drops in a warm drink and take with meals 3 times a day. Millions swear by this tincture (see Amazon for reviews) and I definitely noticed an improvement in my abdominal pain.

12. Incorporate regular light exercise into your lifestyle

- Exercise is critical for a proper functioning gastrointestinal system. It helps regulate bowel movements, releases natural pain killing endorphins and helps alleviate stress. It can include activities such as yoga and walking.

- Exercise at least 30 minutes a day for 5 days a week.

- Try sauna sessions – they are cleansing and rid toxins in your body

13. Stress management

- The gut has its own independent nervous system (enteric), which regulates the processes of digesting foods and eliminating solid waste. The enteric nervous system communicates with the central nervous system and they affect each other. Many IBS sufferers report a high level of stress, which may aggravate bowel symptoms.

- Stress management is vital for IBS sufferers. Massage, yoga, meditation and simple deep breathing exercises can help manage stress levels.

- Rub an oil mixture of peppermint, rosemary and fennel on your abdomen each night to relax your muscles.

- Get enough sleep- at least 7 hours to let your body heal. Nothing will make you anxious and depressed like a chronic sleep debt.

- Consider finding a therapist, if you are struggling to cope and have more serious mental health concerns.

14. Try alternative therapies such as acupuncture

- Doctors studying treatments for IBS have found that an integrated mind body approach, which is common in Eastern medicine, can be effective. Supplement your healing with at least one alternative therapy. It is worth trying, but of course, up to the individual. Some of therapies include hypnosis, acupressure, and cognitive behavioural therapy (CBT). I chose to try acupuncture and had a very positive experience.

- Find a reputable acupuncturist who is trained specifically in digestive complaints. Acupuncture when done correctly helps to resynchronize your organs so they work together in harmony. Not only did it relax me, but it also provided immediate and sustained pain relief.

- Acupuncture also helps in regulating the motility of the digestive tract and in raising the sensory threshold in the gut, which is lowered in IBS sufferers, making them more sensitive to bowel pain and distention.

FINAL THOUGHT

This whole experience has undoubtedly changed me as a person. I feel like I have been to hell and back on this journey, and it has certainly helped me evolve into a deeper, more understanding being and to be grateful for everything that I have, rather than focusing on things that I don't. I no longer complain about trivial things and am just happy to be living a pain free existence.

IBS is a debilitating and lonely illness, and it is paramount that you have unwavering support and access to the right resources to help you overcome it. I could not have gone through this without the encouragement from my wonderful family and partner. Don't ever settle for constantly feeling miserable. You deserve better and don't let others tell you to stop whining, and get on with life.

I believe IBS is curable, however you have to find and treat the underlying cause. Bandaid solutions are only temporary and will have you back at square one feeling even more dejected. Your body is trying to teach you how to get back into balance. Something is out of whack, so you need to listen, find the root cause and treat it for permanent resolution. My secret to healing was prioritizing it. IBS is a puzzle, but not impossible to solve so start now. I hope my story has inspired you to not to give up, to keep searching for relief and ultimately, get your life back.

Printed in Great Britain
by Amazon

ISBN 9781500917821

The Beatitudes...

the blessings from the Sermon on the Mount

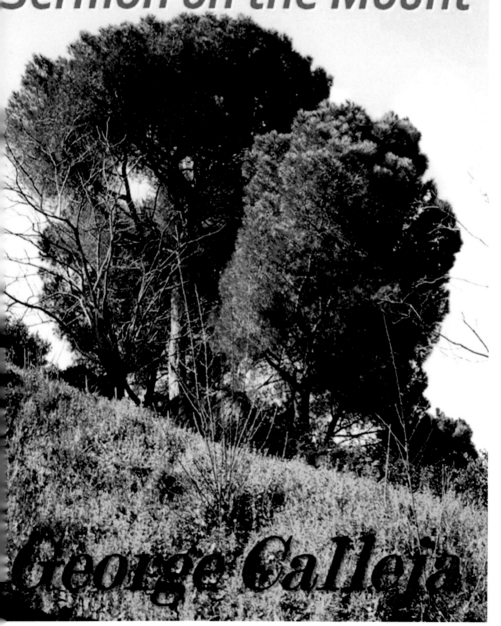

George Calleja